SCHIZOPHRENIA A
SPIRITUAL AWAKENING

Cultural Implications and Implementations

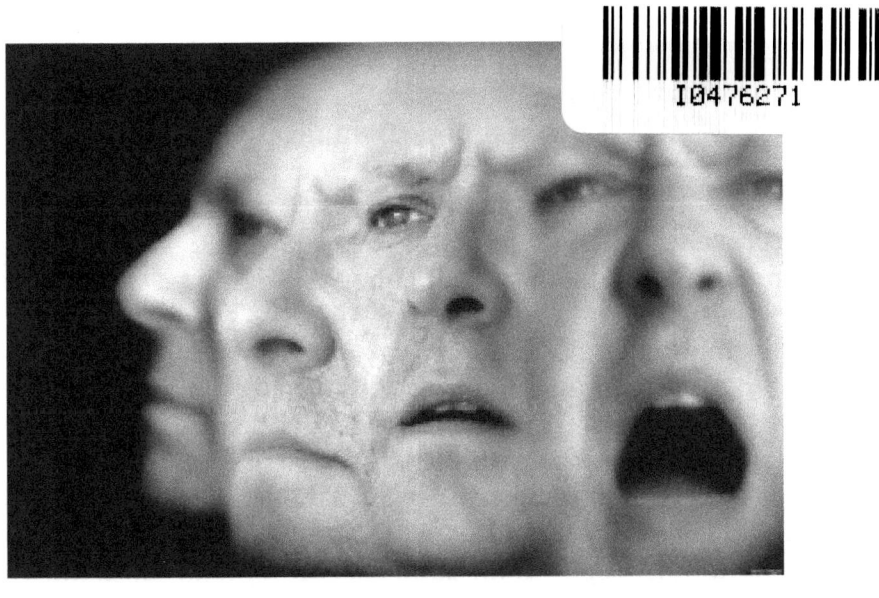

By Patricia A Carlisle

ABOUT THE AUTHOR

Patricia A. Carlisle, MSW, CBT

Patricia Carlisle- A Master Social Worker and a Cognitive Behavioral Therapist (CBT) gives out an expression of how important it is for an individual to take into consideration the concept of self-assessment to know what human, technical and conceptual skills they posses to perform or to achieve what they desire, or to deal with everyday life. However, every particular group of people has their own unique set of ideas, traditions and events including the frame of mind according to which people perform but there are many who faces problems and fail to maintain a healthy mind set affecting their behaviors and performance to those around them.

People like Patricia Carlisle are among those who have felt this urge of serving people and helping them out of their mental crisis towards a healthy life. She has experienced some close encounters in her personal life regarding mental health issues in her family and friends that has encouraged her to pursue this as her career.

Currently Patricia Carlisle is serving as a Certified On-Line Cognitive Behavioral Therapist with an extensive 15years of experience using Cognitive-Behavior Therapy Techniques. She envisions a world where everyone gets mental health treatment with no mental health stigma and to make it real she has already set up her own Holistic Measure Online Comprehensive Behavioral Healthcare Company after retiring from The Nord Center in The Partial Hospitalization Program (PHP) Dept for 5 years and Murtis H. Taylor Mental Health Center as a mental health counselor, psychological support technician and case manager for 10 years to emulsify her skills more professionally. Along with this, she has wrote down her passion as a clinician in 25 or more short books to help individuals and families get their life back, freeing them of the restraints of negative thinking, anxiety and depression by using different approaches. She is highly appreciated among her clients for her flexibility and professionalism of dealing with them graciously.

To reach her, make use of her direct website address: http://therapist2013.wix.com/e-therapy . As she is ready to inspire hope and contribute to health and well-being by providing the best online health care through comprehensive practice, education and research.

Introduction

I want to thank you and congratulate you for choosing the book, *"SCHIZOPHRENIA A SPIRITUAL AWAKENING: Cultural Implications and Implementations"*.

This book contains implications and implementations on how the themes of spirituality and psychotherapy have regularly been dubious in the writing on schizophrenia treatment. A few specialists have contended that religion had no space in the psychotherapy setting given should be grounded in science. Be that as it may, current research shows numerous potential advantages of coordinating issues of religion and spirituality into psychotherapy for people with schizophrenia as to advancing inspiration, wellbeing, flexibility, and cultural parts of one's personality. In the first chapter, suggestions are described for joining spiritual and religious issues in psychotherapy for people with schizophrenia.

Thanks again for choosing this book, I hope you enjoy it!

Table of Contents:

Chapter 1

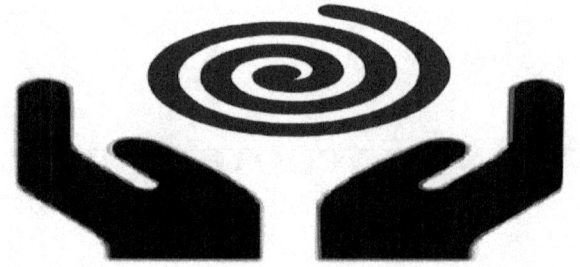

SPIRITUALITY AND PSYCHOTHERAPY

The themes of spirituality and psychotherapy have regularly been dubious in the writing on schizophrenia treatment. A few specialists have contended that religion had contended that religion had no space in the psychotherapy setting given should be grounded in science. Be that as it may, current research shows numerous potential advantages of coordinating issues of religion and spirituality into psychotherapy for people with schizophrenia as to advancing inspiration, wellbeing, flexibility, and cultural parts of one's personality. In this chapter, suggestions are described for joining spiritual and religious issues in psychotherapy for people with schizophrenia. To accomplish this objective, a foundation on the coordination of spirituality into the act of psychotherapy is examined. Next, the writing on spiritually-situated psychotherapy for schizophrenia is given. Clinical ramifications are offered with particular thoughtfulness regarding issues of religious delusions and cultural considerations. Finally, steps for actualizing spiritually situated psychotherapy for people with schizophrenia are portrayed to help suppliers in doing spiritually sensitive consideration.

INCORPORATION OF SPIRITUALITY AND RELIGION

Incorporation of spirituality and religion in psychotherapy practice has been a moderately late advancement. Proficient and experimental brain research amid the twentieth century purposefully rejected issues of religion or spirituality from psychotherapy. In the psychotherapy writing before the 1990s, issues of religion and spirituality would, most every now and again, be recorded in connection to specific sorts of psychopathology, for example, religious delusions in schizophrenia. Additionally, the positive relationship in the middle of religious and spiritual issues and psychological well-being was seldom specified.

Noticeable researchers, for example, Sigmund Freud, John Watson, and Albert Ellis communicated negligible enthusiasm for the study or routine of religion. Truth be told, Freud alluded to religion as a – obsession neurosis and even deliberately dismissed the discord by C.G. Jung, that the limit for religious feeling and symbolism was as essential as sexuality. Regardless of further enthusiasm of significant scholars, for example, William James, Alfred Adler, and Gordon Allport in the association in the middle of spirituality and brain research, the field kept on removing itself from this them.

These researchers implied that psychotherapy practice ought to be grounded in investigative hypothesis and examination. Likewise, the builds of spirituality and religion were not effortlessly quantifiable and did not give themselves enough to such experimental meticulousness. Be that as it may, the previous two decades have seen an ocean of progress in the investigative enthusiasm for religion and spirituality.

Between the years 2000 and 2006, 8,193 articles tending to religion and spirituality from an assortment of hypothetical and observational viewpoints were distributed contrasted with 3,803 such articles distributed throughout sixty years from 1900 to 1959. Yet, little agreement has been come to about how to characterize religion and spirituality and how to recognize one idea from the other. While one conspicuous arrangement of specialists imagine religion as the more extensive term, comprehensive of spirituality, another gathering of researchers perspective spirituality as the more extensive of the two ideas, comprehensive of religion.

In addition, a third gathering of creator's perspective religion and spirituality as particular however covering develops. Here, we hold fast to the more extensive comprehension that religion has a tendency to be related prevalently with institutional representation of the celestial while spirituality has a tendency to be distinguished fundamentally with individual experience of the other worldly.

Religion 2012, 3 84 within the more extensive wellbeing point of view on religion and spirituality, there have been developing endeavors to fuse spiritual viewpoints in the connection of psychotherapy. The thriving enthusiasm for the wellbeing and psychological wellness advantages connected with spirituality and religion may be credited to a few elements.

First the foremost, religion and spirituality have as of lately been set up as imperative inspiring strengths in individuals' lives. Most of the population on the planet sees themselves as being essentially affected by spirituality or religion. Actually, most of the overall population in the United States recognize as spiritual if not religious.

The 2008 American Religious Identification Survey found that very nearly 80% of the population in the United States affirmed to a specific religious connection. This finding was further substantiated by a late Gallup survey where 80% of U.S. inhabitants reported that religion was in any event genuinely imperative in their lives while 54% of the same portrayed religion as being essential.

Second, a collection of late research has noticed some positive effect of spirituality on wellbeing. Over a wide cluster of cultural settings and populaces, religion and spirituality have frequently been discovered to be contributing components to life fulfillment, feeling of individual adequacy, fruitful adapting, and self-regard. Religion and spirituality have been distinguished as imperative figures emotional wellness, incorporating in the recuperation from genuine mental illnesses.

Third, propels in positive brain science as grounded in humanistic and existential intuition moved the center from pathology to sound groups. Constructive brain research is centered on expanding the potential forever pleasure and the advancement of versatility notwithstanding issues or stressors experienced by a man. Basically, the lens of positive brain science moves fare from emotional instability being seen as hurtful and vilifying to following the positive parts of dysfunctional behavior. Mediations are focused on towards wellbeing advancement instead of the treatment and cure of neurotic conditions.

From the viewpoint of upgrade of wellbeing, positive brain science perceives that spirituality, among other positive mental attributes, may develop out of encounters of having a mental illness. The field of positive brain research likewise energizes the experimental investigation of religious and spiritual improvement as contributory component to positive advancement in adulthood. Case in point, spirituality and religiousness are connected with higher-request psychological capacities, which include significance making procedures, moral judgment, and complex critical thinking aptitudes.

Fourth, the development of the field of multicultural advising contextualized in quickly moving cultural patterns, re-incorporated religion and spirituality as focal ideas in psychotherapy rehearse. The multicultural development concentrated on mindfulness and affectability to cultural differences, an imperative part of which is religious and spiritual practice. The development conveyed to light that individuals differ generally on spiritual and religious measurements in pluralistic culture. This group of exploration further enlightened that religious populaces favored spiritually coordinated care over ordinary mental administrations.

At the same time, the moving cultural milieu in the United States in the 1960s and 1970s and huge scale moves in migration achieved expanded familiarity with differences alongside presentation to Eastern religion and reasoning. All the more as of late, mechanical advances in the previous two decades have added to expanded globalization and cultivated expansion in the data trade particularly concerning culture-particular qualities and context oriented variables that add to psychological wellness and prosperity.

These components not just clarify late investigative enthusiasm for comprehension the positive effect of spirituality and religion on wellbeing, additionally underline the benefit of tending to issues of spirituality in psychotherapy with the absolute most difficult emotional wellness conditions.

Chapter 2

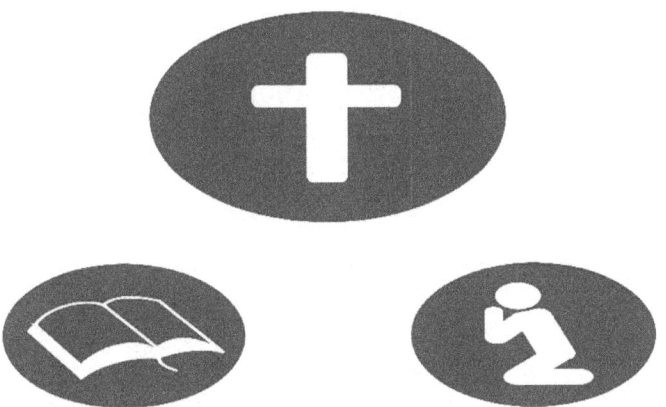

RAMIFICATIONS OF FUSING SPIRITUAL AND RELIGIOUS ISSUES

Here we endeavor to address the ramifications of fusing spiritual and religious issues particularly in the psychotherapy medications of people with schizophrenia.

Numerous meta-analyses have shown that countless methodologies and interventions for the side effects of schizophrenia have been compelling. Then again, the act of psychotherapy for people with schizophrenia has still been disputable in the writing because of inquiries of the adequacy psychotherapy for schizophrenia, particularly in intense cases. Furthermore, the recuperation and recovery model of care people with genuine mental illnesses has regularly neglected the asset of individual psychotherapy.

This oversight may be becomes of the companion bolster center of the recuperation development given the historical backdrop of treacheries conferred by expert suppliers. There are various advantages of psychotherapy for schizophrenia. For one, psychotherapy can give a space to individuals with schizophrenia to investigate their objectives to build life fulfillment while living with emotional instabilities. Some of these objectives incorporate diminishing the effect of the demoralization on self-esteem and feeling good about self, improving versatile adapting systems, and supporting deterrent endeavors to change the course of the ailment.

Also, psychotherapy can encourage the development of a fuller wealthier individual account of recuperation from the disease that is free from shame. Psychotherapy can likewise incorporate the strategy of meta-cognition, i.e., thinking about one's reasoning, to energize and adaptable, element perspective notwithstanding psychosis.

Chapter 3

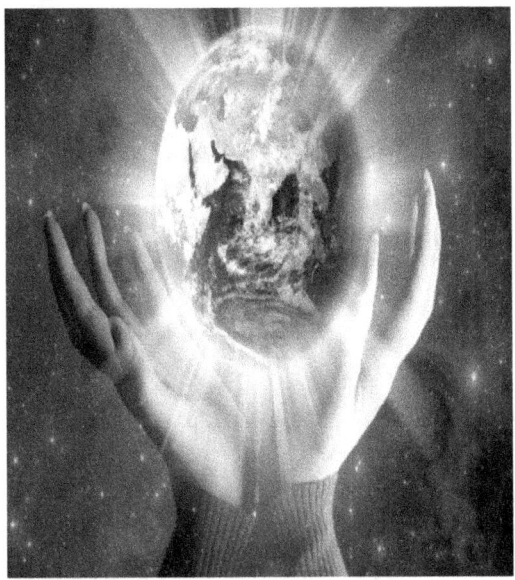

SPIRITUALITY

Spirituality has regularly been recognized as a significant asset for adapting to schizophrenia. Specifically, the recuperation and recovery development has highlighted the essential part of spirituality for the all-encompassing and general working of people influenced by the most incapacitating emotional sicknesses.

The recuperation model is a way to deal with emotional sickness that spotlights on the procedure of carrying on with a wonderful existence of wellbeing and self-governance, instead of the customary treatment concentrate of manifestation disposal. Recuperation from genuine emotional sickness has been introduced as a spiritual process in itself and a trip of confronting spiritual inquiries concerning connections to God, purpose behind the disease, and discovering a place on the planet.

As per few studies, a scope of 30-90% of individuals has reported spirituality and religion to be a standout amongst the most vital parts of recuperation from dysfunctional behaviors. Numerous individual with schizophrenia report an increment of confidence after the utilization of religious adapting and looking for spiritual direction to manage the manifestations of the sickness.

Numerous people have reported and advantage from knowing they can at present have real associations with God in spite of a finding of schizophrenia. Deegan set forth the hypothetical idea that for some individuals in recuperation from schizophrenia, insane musings may even help to get t spirituality. Religion and spirituality are remarkably individual procedures that merit novel consideration regarding the individual story of every individual with schizophrenia.

Individuals with schizophrenia may even characterize their encounters of religion and spirituality uniquely in contrast to each other. Moreover, some exploration recommends that religiousness in people with schizophrenia is illustrative of whatever is left of the populace, albeit religious adapting may be distinctive.

For instance, they may be less participatory in group spiritual occasions, in all probability because of apprehension of shunning. There is an unmistakable significance of incorporating spirituality into recuperation situated treatment models of watched over individuals with schizophrenia.

On the other hand, it is still underrepresented in the recuperation writing and frequently disregarded in clinical consideration. Numerous individuals with schizophrenia don't uncover their religious or spiritual convictions to their suppliers mostly out of apprehension of being marked religiously whimsical and hospitalized automatically.

These discoveries propose the potential advantage of spiritual backings in recuperation arranged treatment to encourage the spiritual training, directing, and practices of individuals with spiritual intrigues who have schizophrenia. Taking into account discoveries from these studies, it is obvious that affectability to spiritual and religious issues in psychotherapy may hold numerous advantages to the person in recuperation from schizophrenia.

Chapter 4

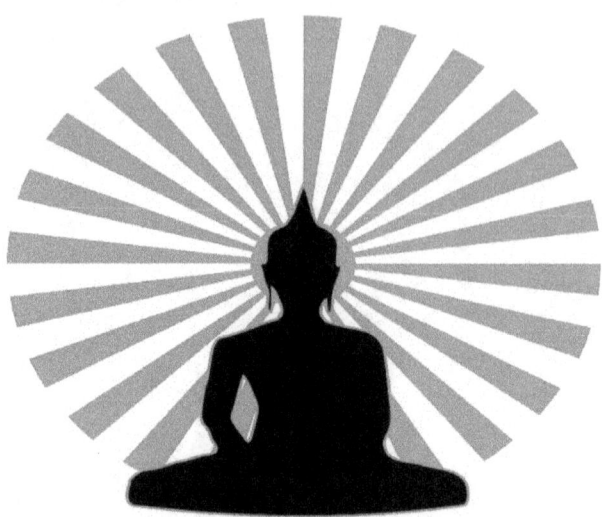

CULTURAL CONSIDERATIONS FOR SPIRITUALLY ORIENTED PSYCHOTHERAPY

Varieties in spiritual and religious practices happen crosswise over ethnic and racial gatherings for people with schizophrenia. Truth be told, adjusting psychological well-being mediations to incorporate the religious and spiritual practices and convictions of a specific cultural gathering is viewed as a culturally capable way to deal with treatment. Some broad contemplation for issues that may emerge when directing spiritually-arranged psychotherapy with schizophrenia will be exhibited here for a few ethnic gatherings.

These contemplations are not intended to be an extensive rundown of every single cultural gathering or religious practices, however some broad cultural contemplations for a few gatherings. Besides, given the extensive level of variety inside of every ethnic gathering, it is vital to comprehend that every individual from these gatherings may not generally fit these rules.

Be that as it may, it can be useful for culturally delicate specialists to be aware of the potential cultural contrasts among people with schizophrenia in regards to religious and spiritual practices. It is likewise vital to note that a large number of the accompanying cultural conventions in spiritual and religious practices may be changed by the procedure of migration.

Chapter 5

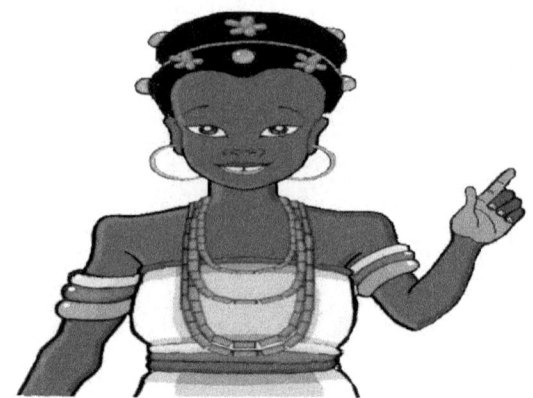

AFRICA

While people of African origin are a heterogeneous gathering with exceptionally various spiritual and religious practices, there are numerous mutual cultural qualities among African Americans specifically because of the historical backdrop of persecution. These regular spiritual qualities incorporated looking for freedom from injustice, and African viewpoints of seeing spirituality inside of all parts of life. Some spiritual and religious practices among African Americans specifically may incorporate the utilization of request of God, the Bible, church participation, religious singing, and the congregation group as adapting methodologies for managing emotional well-being issues in schizophrenia. The congregation has been a site of religious recognition as well as a position of instruction, haven for getting away servitude, monetary assets, and political activism, which permits the congregation to be a profitable asset with different group purposes. Likewise, specialist can consider the association of a spiritual healer or religious pioneer, which is frequently utilized as a part of the treatment of schizophrenia in numerous African and Caribbean conventions.

The themes of spirituality, psychotherapy, and schizophrenia have regularly been uncertain in the writing. Specialists and psychotherapists have generally raised questions as to the suitability of the utilization of spiritual and religious assets in psychotherapy, and have even scrutinized the act of psychotherapy for schizophrenia by and large. Be that as it may, a noteworthy group of writing reflected in here proposes that psychotherapy, and treatment with a spiritual and religious center, can hold numerous advantages for individuals with schizophrenia.

Honing treatment with affectability to parts of religious, spiritual, and cultural differing qualities among people with schizophrenia can further improve this procedure. Distinctive methods applicable to the periods of psychotherapy treatment, for example, preparing, evaluating, arranging, and executing can be considered for incorporating issues of spirituality and religion into treatment in an adaptable however exhaustive way. Consideration of spiritual and religious issues in psychotherapy for people with schizophrenia offers significant chances to give spiritual backing in the person's excursion of reforming.

Chapter 6

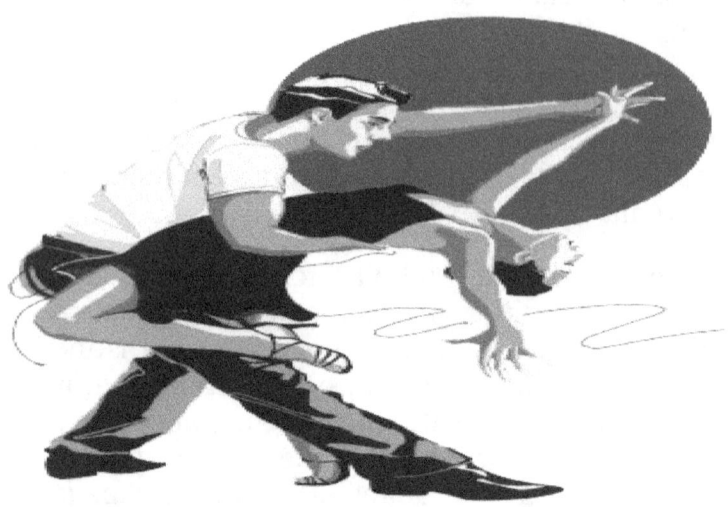

LATIN-AMERICA

Cervantes recommended rules for culturally delicate clinicians to coordinate issues of religion and spirituality into work with people of Latin American plunge. These rules give valuable contemplations to specialists working with Latino people with schizophrenia. Given the extensive variety of assorted qualities in Spanish talking gatherings, there may be huge variety in religious and spiritual practices. Cervantes related the historical backdrop of indigenous Latin American bunches whose religious and spiritual practices were annihilated by colonizers and supplanted with Europe and conventions that blended indigenous practices with Christian and Catholic religions.

Along these lines, numerous Latino clients may watch Christianity, Catholicism, indigenous religions, or some mix. The indigenous commitment to religious practices of Latino people may be introduced in love of divinities and hallowed places, reverential offerings, request to God, and journeys. Mestizo spirituality among Mexican aggregates specifically may reflect religious values in differing qualities and connectedness to the social and physical environment.

Cervantes stressed that mix of Latino spirituality and religious practices is fundamental for successful psychotherapy.

For specialists working with people with schizophrenia of Latin American plunge, affectability to these religious and spiritual practices and convictions can improve a culturally harmonious wellspring of backing.

Chapter 7

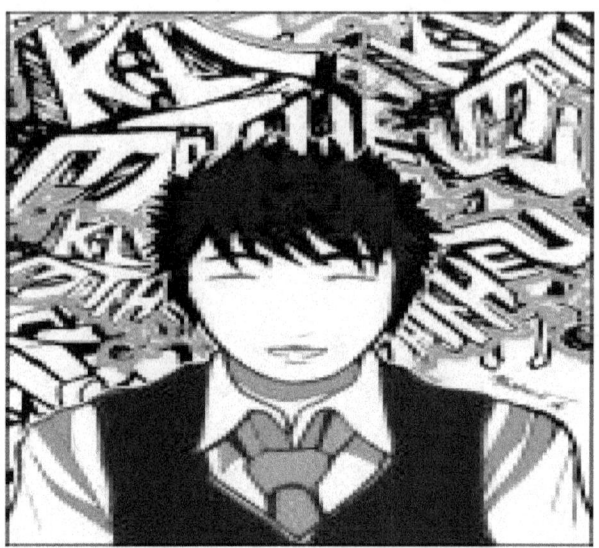

ASIAN

While the Asian continent is comprised of a diverse array of religions and religious practices, some of the most commonly practiced religions are outlined in this section. Researchers presented guide lines for clinicians working with Asian clients of diverse Hindu, Buddhist, and Islamic backgrounds that have implications of psychotherapy with individuals with schizophrenia. Hinduism and Buddhism involve meditation practices that can be incorporated into therapy to reduce anxiety and distress that often accompanies psychotic symptoms.

For example, the Svetasvatara Upanishad meditation in Hindu practices or the walking meditation and mindfulness exercised in Buddhist meditation may be integrated into therapy to reduce the anxiety, impulsivity, and distress often associated with psychotic symptoms. These authors suggested that in the case of Islamic religions, spiritual values of benevolence, personal development, and forgiveness can promote positive religious coping in therapy for individuals with schizophrenia.

In addition, Islamic mysticism, namely, Sufism, provides more detailed psychological perspectives on mental health which foster growth through the use of dance, music, meditation and prayer, and may also hold utility in mental health treatment for individuals with schizophrenia.

Chapter 8

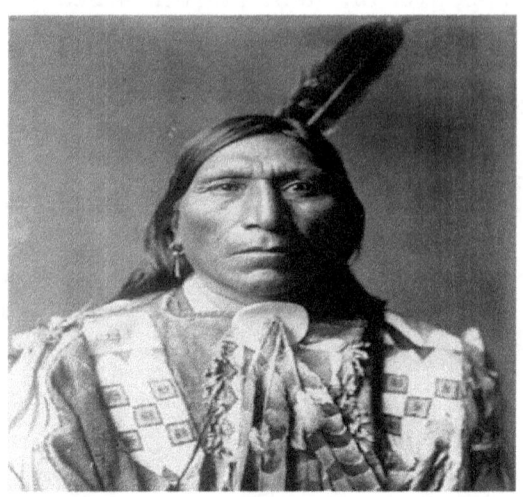

NATIVE AMERICAN

There is an extensive level of assorted qualities crosswise over tribal gatherings inside of Native American cultures. Numerous Native American gatherings don't fragment spirituality from whatever is left of everyday life, yet rather give a spiritual mixture for the duration of day by day life and culture. Some tribal gatherings at first saw insane like states as having a spiritual worth to the culture. In any case, the impact of Western qualities has driven numerous Native American gatherings to come to see emotional sickness as additionally demonizing.

Also, Europe a colonization additionally conveyed Christianity to numerous Native American bunches. Affectability to the distinctive spiritual logic and potential Western impacts on religion are imperative contemplations for the specialist working with a person with schizophrenia of Native American plunge.

Culturally delicate psychotherapy with people with schizophrenia may mean adjusting oneself to the singular's religious or spiritual personality to work towards a coveted objective, conduct, disposition, or enthusiastic state.

Clinicians ought to additionally practice alertness and think about religious counter-transference, including familiarity with inclination towards the customer's religion because they could call their own religious or spiritual practices, or maybe distrust toward religion and spirituality altogether.

Conclusion

Thank you again for choosing this book!

I hope this book was able to help you to understand how spirituality and religious practices can help individuals with schizophrenia.

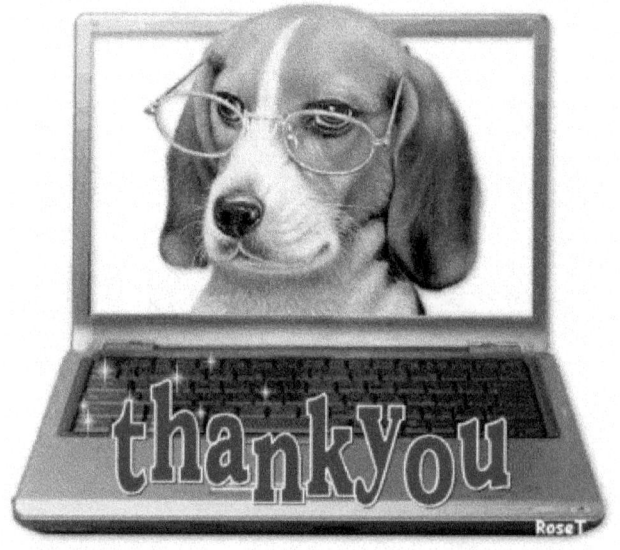

Finally, if you enjoyed this book would you be kind enough to leave a review for this book on Amazon? It'd be greatly appreciated!

Thank you and good luck!

Preview Of 'The Depression Cure: How to overcome depression and become depression free'

Chapter 1
MOOD DISORDER IS DEPRESSION
Tackling depression head-on the right way

Recovery begins when we overcome depression and become totally depression free. Treatment for depression begins when one analyses the causes and learns the symptoms of depression. Depression cure needs much patience on the part of the patient and the physician. Depression unlike sadness and happiness is not a normal human emotion. Naturally, many people do not realize they are depressed and let this ailment go unnoticed. However, it is because there is every possibility for this serious mood disorder to cause disruptions to normal social life and even death, one need to look at the signs. When you feel lonely listless and down-in-the-dumps, you take a walk or have a refreshing drink and you feel bright and cheerful once again. In those situations when you feel that your thoughts and feelings, your sense of well being seem to have disappeared, gone on a vacation, you have to sit up and straighten your tie. Depression cure unlike relief from stress does not happen naturally.

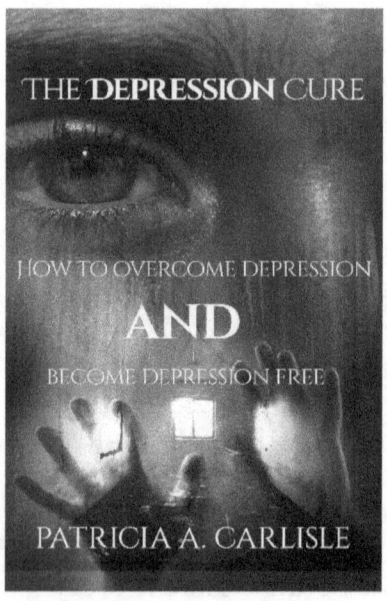

To learn more about (The Depression Cure: How To Overcome Depression and Become Depression Free) go to amazon.com

Check Out My Other Books

Below you'll find some of my other popular books that are popular on Amazon and Kindle as well. Alternatively, you can visit my author page on Amazon to see other work done by me.

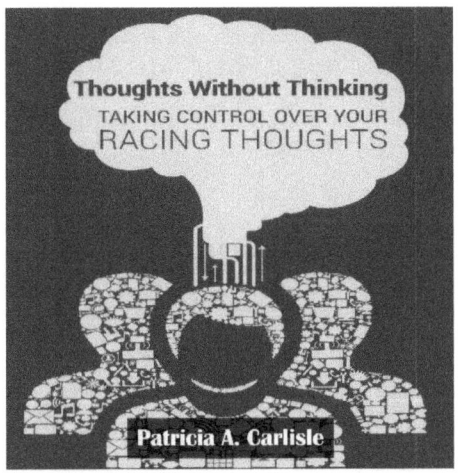

Thoughts Without Thinking: Taking control over your racing thoughts.

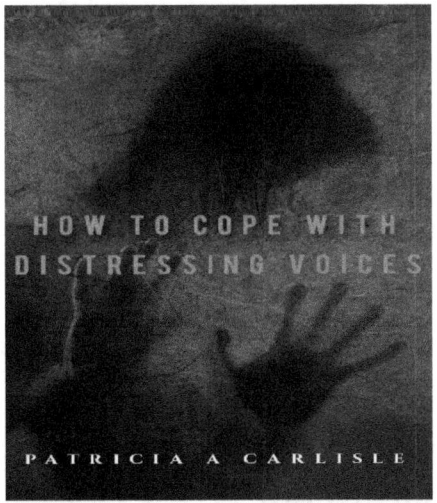

How to cope with distressing voices.

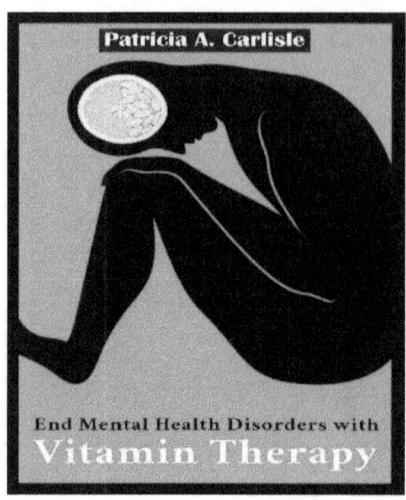

End Mental Disorders with vitamin therapy.

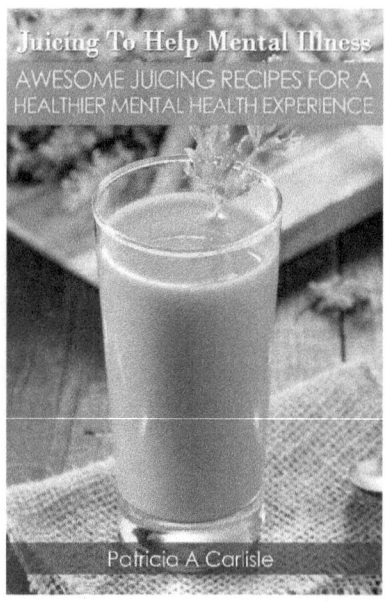

Juicing to Help Mental Illness: Awesome juicing recipes for a healthier mental health.

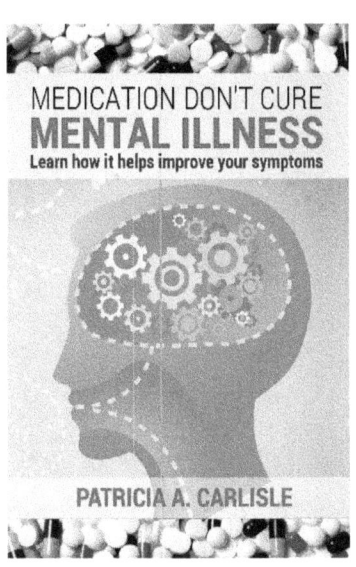

**MEDICATION DON'T CURE MENTAL ILLNESS:
Learn how it helps improve your symptoms.**

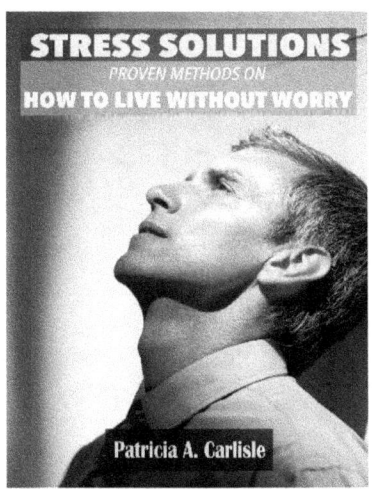

**STRESS SOLUTIONS: Proven methods on how to live
without worry.**

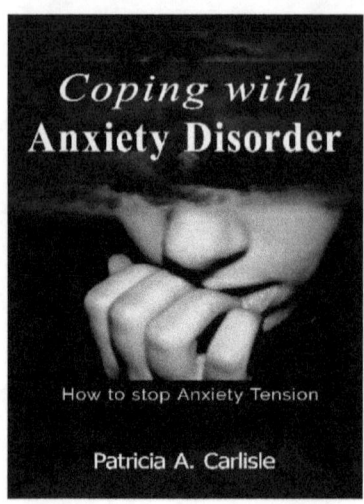

Coping with Anxiety Disorder: How to stop Anxiety Tension.

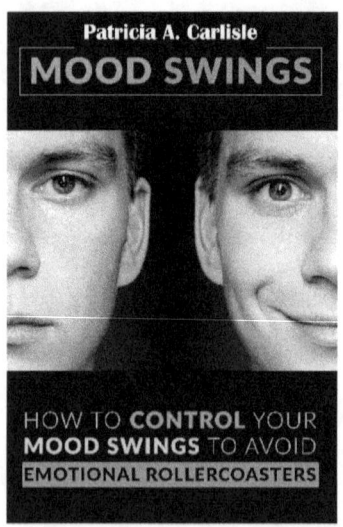

Mood Swings: How to control your mood swings to avoid emotional rollercoster's.

BONUS: SUBSCRIBE TO THE FREE BOOK

Beginners Guide to Yoga & Meditation

"Stressed out? Do You Feel Like The World Is Crashing Down Around You? Want To Take A Vacation That Will Relax Your Mind, Body And Spirit? Well this Easy To Read Step By Step

E-Book Makes It All Possible!"

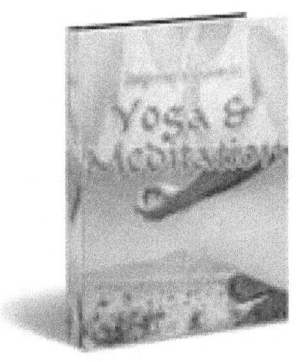

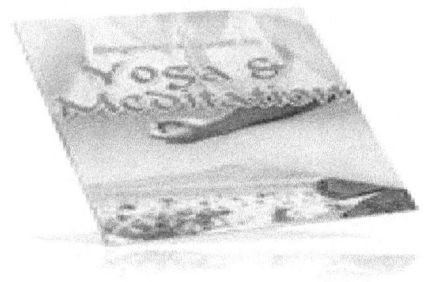

Instructions on how to join our mailing list, and receive a free copy of "Yoga and Meditation" can be found in any of my Kindle eBooks.

NOTES

NOTES

NOTES

NOTES

NOTES